IN SEARCH OF
ADVENTURE

IN SEARCH OF ADVENTURE

Short stories about women who cycle

RUTH MCINTOSH

Maryam Amatullah, Melanie Carroll, Susan Doram, Snjezana Jojic, Liane Higham, Indigo Kelly-Forest, Sarah Layden, Janine Morrall, Janet Steel, Joanne Westwood, Nicky Woods

Good Apple Copy for Slow-Cycle

CONTENTS

All of the women who have contributed their stories to this book spend time supporting other women.

They are advocates for wider participation in cycling, women's health and much more.

Thank you for being brilliant.

Ruth

Introduction

I was chatting to a friend the other day who asked me, "What do you want these stories about women who cycle to achieve?" I gave it some thought and it's this: I want to thank all of the wonderful people who have passed on their passion for cycling to me and to share my love of the freedom I feel when I'm on a bike.

Imagine how chuffed I was when my sister told me that she and her friend had cycled from West London to Bath to celebrate her 50th birthday after reading the draft of my book! This was their first tour on their bikes. They hadn't been sure if they, or their bikes, were up to scratch until I reassured them that they certainly were. They might have done it anyway but it's great to think that I made a difference.

I understand all too well that it's not always easy to get going. Actually, the idea for this book only started when I found myself with time on my hands whilst recovering from Coronavirus. My bike was languishing in a dusty garage and I needed something else to cheer me up.

Inspiration came to me during a Zoom call with some friends I had made during a cycling holiday. It was just the thing I needed to set the wheels in motion. I've always wanted to write about women and to get our voices heard. Lockdown seemed like the perfect opportunity to take on a storytelling project.

Soon eleven other women were on board and I had transcribed their stories in full. The final stories have been edited but the words remain their own, just as every woman told me her story.

I learned a lot through their experiences. Most started on basic bikes; there were times when they doubted themselves and they all had to deal with some difficult stuff. Many had also coped with one or more health conditions: arthritis, brain injury, diabetes, excess weight, heart problems, fatigue and thyroid problems. One or two had fallen off their bicycles then got back on them to recover. I felt really lucky listening to their stories and they inspired me to start cycling more regularly again.

My hope is that sharing these stories will inspire anyone who is dreaming of getting on a bike, joining a cycling initiative or planning adventures of their own.

CHAPTER 1

Maryam Amatullah

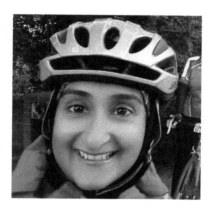

Maryam lives in Leicester and her journey in cycling has taken her from being stuck indoors with her daughter in the summer holidays to being an inspirational cycling leader and one of Cycling UK's 100 women in cycling. She's shy but she's got a fiery side to her, especially when she's climbing hills or dealing with inconsiderate drivers! Through training others to ride as a volunteer, Maryam was chosen to be an Olympic Dove which involved performing in the 2012 Opening Ceremony.

3

MARYAM'S STORY

In 2010, I was starting to exercise gently after being unwell for a few years due to hypothyroidism. My eleven year old daughter was just sitting on the PlayStation most of the day in the summer holidays. It was really bugging me that she was indoors and not getting outside. I thought, "I've got to do something for her and something for myself as well," so I looked around and got myself a mountain bike. We explored our local surroundings, starting at the park, then we went from park to park and then a bit further afield. She got more confident and shot up hills while I was huffed and puffed behind, not even half way up! I really enjoyed our time together and it had a positive effect on my health. Later, when she was in Year 8, it wasn't "cool" any more so it was just me on my own!

Where I live is predominantly Asian and Muslim. You didn't see any women cycling around here, none at all, no matter what colour. I certainly didn't notice any. An Asian Muslim woman on a bike? You just didn't see it here. I was turning heads and it was making me feel uncomfortable, especially as I wear a head-covering so I stood out even more. Some of the guys that worked in the local shops would stand on the corner with their arms folded. I thought, "Oh no! Do I have to go past them?" I'd get home a bit tearful and would dread going out.

Nevertheless, I was determined to continue. I kept telling myself, "They're only looking because they want to cycle too."

I had been on some local Sky Rides and wanted to be part of a women's group but I didn't know any. I contacted the council who put me in touch with Elizabeth Barner at CTC/ Cycling UK to find out if they had any groups. They said, "Why don't you set something up? We'll train you up as a cycling instructor." My journey started from there working on various projects delivering training to adults and children for the city council and independently. I ran a project in the summer holidays for women in the community with children and it was more successful than I thought it would be with twenty five women and their children turning up.

Ten years on, I don't feel self-conscious anymore. I am much more confident than what I used to be. That dreaded feeling of going outside the front door thinking, "I just can't face them today" is old news. Today, when I was coming back from my bike ride with my friend Yasmin, I saw five Asian women on their bikes cycling through the park. It always makes me smile. Women have begun to ride. It's had a knock-on effect and it's growing, like a snowball effect. One person does it, so it encourages somebody else to do it then it increasingly gets bigger. A lot more people are cycling since lockdown and it's making the news. People are wanting to get back on a bike or wanting to learn.

I never imagined myself cycle touring. When my friend Susan won some accommodation for a cycle holiday in Somerset, she took a few of us with her. We spent three nights in an old coach house so we could spend our days riding the Cheddar Gorge and the hills, even though I hate hills!

After that Susan was badgering us to do the Coast-to-Coast. I said, "No, I can't do it!" mainly because the route goes through the Lake District and I know those killer hills! Susan is a strong rider, I'm nowhere as good as her, I can just about get up Leicestershire hills. I had already written myself off. Susan carried on asking, so I said, "If Lindsey does it, I'll do it" because I knew that we were about the same pace. Lindsey said, "I'll do it... if Liz does it" so three of us agreed that we'd do it at a manageable pace and go along with Susan. We were really excited. We didn't do any special training because we were already commuting. Two weeks before the trip we started loading up our panniers a bit more. Since then, we've done a tour every year and continued what Susan started.

I do the cycling projects, getting more women to ride and building their confidence, mainly because I like helping other women. I want them to discover the fun of being on two wheels, how they can easily get around the city and explore their local environment. It's good for health and mood boosting, it's environmentally friendly. We get women who have never sat on the bike, who are really scared. I love the positive benefits I get out of it, watching people smile and that exhilaration as they start to pedal for the first time and the joy on their face. It's just magic you come home and think, "This is just brilliant, they've learnt a new skill for life." I love what I do but it's them: they put the effort in, I'm just talking.

I get it now. I understand why new starters are nervous. I went on a BMX course and got a bit of an insight into how they might feel because I had to take risks and I was worried that I might break a bone. My eyes were popping out of my head and I thought: "This is how new learners feel!" I am always extra sensitive at work with women who may have had health problems or mental issues or really low confidence because I understand where they're coming from.

I've always found myself to be my own biggest barrier. I don't believe in myself and my abilities and that holds me back from saying, "I'm going to go ahead and do that." It's nice when you're part of a group because we're all inspiring each other. We all have a story to tell and we all get motivated by each other. That's what I love about being part of a female group or club it's that we've all got something to offer. Because I'm a shy person, cycling makes me feel very different, it makes me feel more confident when I'm on the bike. I think it's maybe something to do with the chemicals being released?

Most of all, on cycle tours, there is a sense of achievement. It's an adventure that I have done by myself, something away from my kids and my husband, something personal for me.

Having the time to free the mind and to do your own thing, being yourself. It's that Me, Myself and I moment! And my relationship with hills? That's changed. Doing the Coast to Coast has helped me to embrace hills: they're an important part of the journey!

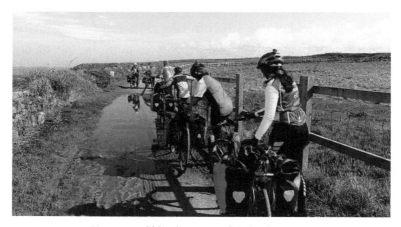

Maryam and friends on one of their adventures

It's nice when you're part of a group because we're all inspiring each other. We all have a story to tell and we all get motivated by each other.

Maryam Amatullah

CHAPTER 2

Melanie Carroll

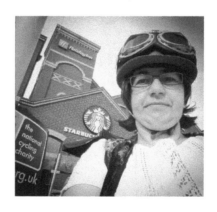

Melanie rides an e-bike called Tolkein which takes her on adventures in and around Lincoln. It's a sit-up-and-beg e-bike with a chimp mascot and basket in pride of place because Melanie is a great believer in allowing people to do their own thing. Indeed, she's a great spokesperson for helping people of all ages and abilities to find the courage to get on bikes. This woman CAN but she also understands the kind of self-talk that plagues us and stops us from believing that cycling is for everyone.

MELANIE'S STORY

I had a heart defect when I was a little kid. My mum used to pull me along on a tricycle rather than putting me in a pushchair to go to school which wouldn't have looked so good at that age. My love for bikes started from that because that was how I got to and from everywhere. As I got older and better and stronger I was finally able to get on my own two wheels and pedal myself.

As an adult I cycled to work for years until we had some really bad winters about 10 years ago. I realised that if I took the bus I could do some reading, and I love reading, hence why I own a bookshop. For 3 ½ years I never got on my bike then they put their bus ticket up by £1.50! I thought, "Wait a minute, I've got my bike why am I not cycling?" I fell back in love with it.

About seven years ago I saw an advert for Sky Ride leaders and I said to my mum, "I really like the idea of that but I don't think that I'm a good enough cyclist." My mum said, "You've been cycling all your life, I'm pretty sure you're a good enough cyclist... all you need to do is give it a go."

I sent off to do the course and the day before I thought, "I'll be the only one on a sit up and beg, I don't have any qualifications to do this." I was sitting in a café and my mum bought me a cycle chimp which is now my mascot. My mum said, "Put the chimp on your basket, the chimp can be your mascot and you can shut up the chimp in your head."

At the training I was the only one with a sit up and beg bike, and the only one of two women. We were asked to introduce ourselves. I said, "I am Melanie and I'm the rider with the chimpcycle!" and everybody laughed. After that I was OK. We went out and cycled and I realised that I was as qualified as any of them. Actually, I was quite capable.

A lot of the adults I have trained through Bikeability have been older women who came from households where there wasn't a lot of money or where cycling was seen as something that their brothers did, not what they did so they never learned to cycle. They had husbands who could cycle and grown-up kids who could cycle but they never learned as young girls. Because they were now at retirement age, they wanted to be able to spend more time with the family, but most of the family were cycling.

The best one I ever had was a 78 year-old woman who had never cycled before. She was relatively fit and showed up with an electric bike which she'd been out and bought for herself. Her husband had recently died and so she needed some way to get out and about locally. Her children and grand-children were cyclists on the weekends so she booked a course to learn to cycle. She even wheeled it out of the car, she didn't even ride it to the centre and said, "How do I get on this thing love?" I said, "This one's easy sweetheart, you just step over." By the end of two hours, we'd got her cycling around the car park. Not brilliantly, don't get me wrong: she was not ready to go out on any roads by any stretch of the imagination. I said to her, "If you go out on cycle paths, can you ensure that they're a bit empty?" It took time to build up that smile on her face but it's something that I'll never forget.

People tend to be very tense at first so I get all my newbies to laugh. You know how Woody Woodpecker laughs? He he he he he! When you get tense, you need to laugh like Woody Woodpecker to loosen your muscles up and let everything go. Just do the floppy dance. It makes people think I'm absolutely nuts but it breaks the ice makes them laugh and that's the important bit. You've got to enjoy it you've got to relax into it even though it's scary because you're learning. Most people are peddling within two hours and they need to acknowledge their achievements.

Self-talk is really important. Absolutely doubting yourself is a recurring theme in all of the groups that I teach. Sometimes they go into it with a mantra of, "I can't: I'm not good enough." They can and they are good enough. We need to stop comparing ourselves to everybody else.

My mum was a really strong woman who told me that I could do anything, but the rest of society secretly tells you as a young girl, "You can't do that: that's what other people do... it's what blokes do." Changing that only takes one of us with conviction. It can spread like a germ, and I want it to become as virulent as Covid so women begin to get out there and cycle.

So many women think they can't. I have conversations with women on a weekly basis who say, "I couldn't do that." I've got two spare bikes in my garage and I always offer them up. Sometimes it takes them five times to build up the courage but if we keep having those conversations and making that offer available then people reach a point when they are not joking and take action.

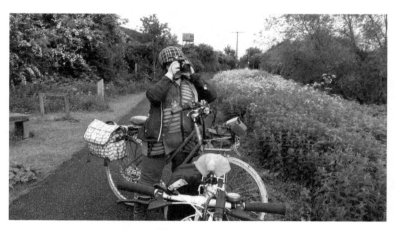

Melanie taking pictures along the way

All of my bikes have a chimp attached to them. The chimp owns the bike, I'm just the chimp's rider. I make up little stories about the adventures we have. They're not really adventures, they're just longer journeys that we take home and I spin them into bits of stories.

My current bike is named Tolkein because of the adventures that we go on. It's the chimp that gets into the adventures, I'm only ever the rider so it's never my fault! It's always the chimp on the bike that causes the problem.

When you get tense, you need to laugh
like Woody Woodpecker, he-he-he-he-he
to loosen your muscles up and let
everything go!

Melanie Carroll

CHAPTER 3

Susan Doram

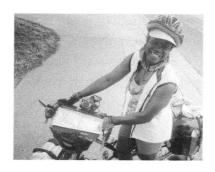

Susan returned to living in Leicester just before lockdown having just completed a 2½-year-long trip around the world. One of the brilliant things about Susan's trip is the way that she embraced serendipity. Although Susan travelled on her own, she wasn't always alone. People were more friendly along the way because she was a single woman. This gave her an opportunity to make friendships with other women, giving her unique access and insights into life behind closed doors in many different countries. Susan has featured in Cycling UK's list of 100 women in cycling, she's a key member of Leicester Women's Velo and a radio regular with a great laugh!

SUSAN'S STORY

Planning and de-cluttering in preparation for my World Trip took two years. One of the biggest things was getting my cat re-homed. I gave that cat the best years of my life! I was working full time at that point so I could save some money. Afterwards, I realised that I could have gone earlier if I'd not spent so much time worrying about the cat, saving and de-cluttering the things I didn't necessarily need. There was a lot of clutter. When I was 18 and got a gold crown, the dentist said, "Maybe you might want a plaster cast of your teeth?" so I carried the impression of that around with me for years from house to house! Having said that, a lot of the planning was making sure that I had the right Visas. I also prepared extra paperwork, proving that I had a house in the UK, and copies of vaccination certificates.

I flew to Vancouver first and cycled the west coast of Canada and the USA. I then travelled to Hawaii, New Zealand, Tonga, Australia, Indonesia, Singapore, Malaysia, Thailand, Cambodia, Vietnam, Taiwan, South Korea, Portugal and Spain. I know it sounds like a lot but I was away for a long time! Some people visit more countries and visit the whole of the country but for me it wasn't ticking off destinations on a list, it was the whole experience. I never did more than sixty miles, ideally thirty a day. I think in my first year I did less mileage than I'd been doing at home in the UK.

The whole beauty of cycle touring is that it takes you off the beaten track. Some places draw you in and people are surprised when you go back to have breakfast in the same place for two days in a row. Websites like Warmshowers and Couch-surfing make it easier to find somewhere to stay. I prefer Warmshowers because it is run by and for cyclists. On the Couchsurfing website there are boxes you can tick to choose your preferences. There's tick-boxes: "male or female?" They also give information about where you'll sleep: "Shared surfaces" being one of the options! I got a marriage proposal in Thailand but that was just a marriage of convenience. I met some guy in Cambodia who was really friendly and I didn't realise that he maybe wanted more until he had to spell it out. A lot of people would feed me and pay the bill because they're curious. In a lot of cases it's general hospitality as I am a guest in their country. They'd often ask: "Where do you come from?" "How old are you?" "Where's your husband?" I remember being asked that last one by a five-year old!

Interestingly, things had changed in Tonga. I was there 25 years ago when you wouldn't see a Tongan woman out in the street on her own, she had to be chaperoned. The chaperones could be quite brutal. If a girl went to a disco, she would have to be chaperoned. If a boy asked a girl to dance and was too persistent, you'd see the chaperones hitting the boys and telling them to go away. It isn't like that anymore, and so many more women were driving and out and about on their own.

I met a young woman in the USA called Clara who cycled across the States from East to West. I met her in Oregon. She'd got some interesting stories about her experiences in Middle America. She stayed at people's houses and asked if she could put her tent in their garden and they'd invite her in to stay in a bed. They reasoned that if they had a daughter, they would want her to be looked after. She started her journey with a chap who was Latino-American but they parted ways. I remember her saying that she thought he would struggle to get the same kind of reception.

In Malaysia and Vietnam young people want to travel but their parents won't let them. I met a young man in Vietnam, he was a Warmshowers host, and he started doing it to introduce his parents to people: it was his way of getting permission. It's hard for young people, especially if they work in the family business because there's no choice. This is particularly the case for the Chinese-Malaysians who've had family businesses for generations.

Some people and places are easier to get to know than others. I went to Thailand twice and the second time I stayed for six months. Part of the reason was to get to know the people and their culture. I was working as a teacher and one day on my way to work I saw a very large gazebo which had a coffin in it with a picture of the deceased on the wall outside somebody's house. The gazebo was there for quite a few days. I was curious to find out what happened at Thai funerals. It was really odd because none of my Thai work colleagues were very forthcoming with information. I asked the foreign teachers who taught at the school if they knew about this tradition. They didn't know and they didn't seem particularly interested. In contrast, my experience in Tonga was the complete opposite; I was told all about their culture, stories and traditions. For example, if you are a woman and your mother dies you cut your hair off and give it to the matriarch of the family.

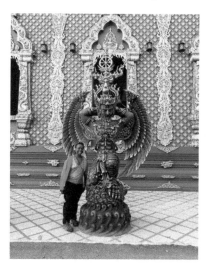

The Blue Temple, Chiang Rai, Thailand

I was overwhelmed by people's generosity. When I was in Tonga there was a cyclone. It was pretty wild, the worst cyclone for sixty years. I was staying with a friend and she had given me the best bed because I was the honoured guest. During the cyclone I was in the bedroom and the rest of the family were in the living room together. Things were being blown about. A coconut could have blasted through the window and knocked me out! By the end of the night I was in the living room with everyone else because my bed had been under the window. Safety in numbers! There was very little damage to the house. Luckily my friend's husband was a competent carpenter.

Speaking English is a big advantage. Most people would talk to me in English. It is a bit embarrassing really isn't it? South Korea was the place where I struggled most with not being able to speak or recognise any of the language. I had taken a picture dictionary with me so I could point to that but I didn't use it much. A lot of people are amazed that tourists like me visit their country and they'll go out of their way to help, especially if you're a woman.

Passport control is always a stress. My heart's beating in my chest. I think: "Am I going to get stopped this time?" On this tour I went to the USA twice. In 2017 people said, "We're glad you've come to visit... we hope you see that the States is not like it is portrayed on the TV". I stayed on the west coast, which is far more liberal-minded. Lots of the American people who I met along the way weren't happy with the way things were going.

Two years later, in November 2019, when I arrived back in the USA for the second time, I was detained for 5 hours. It wasn't nice to know the only reason I was being stopped was because of the colour of my skin. I had to wait in a room with about 100 other people and there was not one white person waiting in that room.

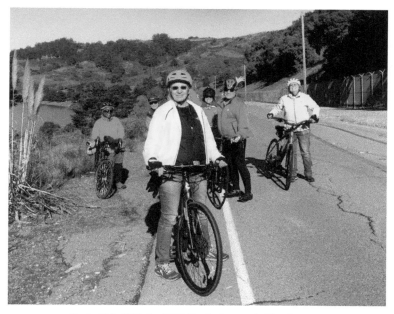

Cycle Ride With the PMS Cycle Group, California, USA

Originally I was going south from Vancouver, Canada all the way down to the bottom of South America but I ended up going west instead because I couldn't resist the pull of Polynesia. Listening to advice along the way, I erred on the side of caution and went to countries which were safer. When you read other people's blogs, they're often about hardship. That didn't appeal to me. Although I planned for the trip, I didn't have a fixed itinerary and made it up along the way.

I guess I like communing with people more than nature! I ride my bike with a blue tooth speaker so there's not going to be any birdsong! Favourite artists to cycle to are Luther Vandross and Stevie Wonder so I share a little bit of Luther and Stevie everywhere I go!

Susan Doram

CHAPTER 4

Liane Higham

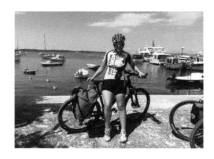

Looking at Liane, you wouldn't know that she's faced potentially debilitating health problems and that a lot of her cure has been a positive mental attitude (sheer bloody-mindedness) and getting on a bicycle. A former pioneer of Breeze in Northamptonshire, Liane is a passionate advocate for getting young people and women involved in cycling for pleasure, commuting and communing with nature. Liane now lives in Sydney and works as a Cycling Instructor.

LIANE'S STORY

For my 40th birthday, my husband booked for us to go on holiday. He booked mountain-biking, his interest, in Greece. On mountains! I saw Greece as a holiday place, beaches and sunshine. It was not that! It was full-on rock descents avoiding goats. There was a lot of climbing and the bike that I took out was a hard-tail, so it only had front suspension and not much of it at that. We had quite an interesting journey. There was a lot of swearing! There was a lot of screaming at goats to get out of the way! I only had one working brake so I didn't have a lot of stopping power. Although I swore a lot, peed a little and was very scared, I came away with a love of mountain biking.

At that stage I was only riding off-road, across country on canal towpaths to the coffee shop. It was only seeing a bike that was so beautiful that got me hooked. It was very clever of the bike shop to loan me the bike, (Reader, I bought it!) I really enjoyed nipping out on a Saturday morning and doing 45 miles to the coffee shop. My sons were older so we could enjoy cycling together as a family. We went to Trail Centres like Cannock Chase, Swinley Forest and Bike Park Wales.

I was still working in sales in an office. I used to put the bike downstairs but the company decided for Health and Safety reasons, it had to be outside, it couldn't be in the building. On the third time I locked it up outside, it was stolen. Someone came in a van, blocked the view from the office window and cut the bike lock. I was upset about the bike being stolen and the management's attitude, that I should've had a cheaper bike. When I reported it to the Police, they were unconcerned but suggested that I shouldn't be commuting on that route. I had a discussion with my husband, who was working in Australia at the time, and he suggested that I quit. So I did, taking the summer off to spend time with my children.

I started riding more and met some women who were discussing Breeze. I was like, "Wow! This is great I'd really love to do this." I contacted Breeze and they said, "The nearest we've got is Leicester because Northamptonshire's really not a cycling county." I said, "I'd really like to launch in Northamptonshire." I rounded up my friends and said, "You have to come on a bike ride with me!" then I advertised it wider on Facebook.

I knew some traffic-free routes through woods, along canal towpaths. I contacted my local Council and the lady in sport there was really keen on getting more women into cycling. She did flyers for me and supported the initiative. Breeze Northamptonshire was born!

There were so many opportunities in British Cycling at that time, going to the velodrome and riding with Breeze. Having never cycle-camped, and knowing nobody else who was doing it, I signed up to the Women's French Adventure with Indigo Kelly-Forest. I thought, "I want to do this for me now, I want a week away." I could only take one week off from family life to do something purely for me. It felt pretty selfish but it was fantastic. I would not have done it if I was completely on my own.

To me cycling has always been freedom. At the age of seventeen, I was diagnosed with rheumatoid arthritis. I was told it would be debilitating, that I would never have children and I would probably end up in a wheelchair. Doctors don't really understand how it triggers or how it will end up but cycling gave me the peace of mind and kept me active. I'm in my mid fifties now and, last August, I finally had a double hip replacement with titanium in both femurs because I had no cartilage left. When I saw the surgeon, I said, "I can ride a bike but I can't walk to the bus stop." He was amazed that I could even get on a bike. Freedom from pain is freedom from so many things. It often isn't understood how older people can cycle, but they can. It's amazing to see how many people a bicycle enables, even people who struggle with walking.

Coming to Sydney, people said, "You can't ride a bike here... it's too dangerous." Until you find your tribe you don't realise there are some areas of the city where it's really normal, there are cargo bikes and kids on bikes. Maybe there's something about women of a certain age who don't like being told, "You can't!" I think, "I can!" And I do!

When I was in the UK, a year before I came to Australia in 2016, I had these awful headaches. I couldn't work out if I was menopausal. I didn't know what was the matter with me. I was waking up in the middle of the night shaking with pain. After a while, I got an appointment with a specialist. The specialist did an MRI scan and said, "I'm sorry, I suspect a brain tumour and it's really invasive." I was referred to Oxford and given a diagnosis of two months to live.

I like proving doctors wrong. I was advised not to drive. I said, "I use a bike for transport." The doctor was concerned about me having seizures and said that I couldn't ride on my own. I spent six months in and out of Oxford, seeing six different brain surgeons. They never did another MRI and my surgery got delayed three times.

The second time it got cancelled, the Breeze Champions ride was on in Warwickshire. I argued that I was feeling fine. I managed to get leave from hospital and did the Breeze 100km challenge with a fantastic team around me. When the Macmillan nurse checked in the next day she said, "How was it?" I said, "Fantastic, yeah it was 100km". She said, "I thought you meant about 5 miles!"

When I was waiting for the awake surgery, I got asked if I would take part in an MRI scan for a research project using a new machine. They were using the equipment to look for brain tumours in children. The next day the surgeon said, "The tumour is gone, it's not there so we're not going to do the surgery." Had they done it and cut me open, they would have cut out the parts of my brain that would have affected movement, memories and speech. I would have been in recovery for years. Always agree to medical research!

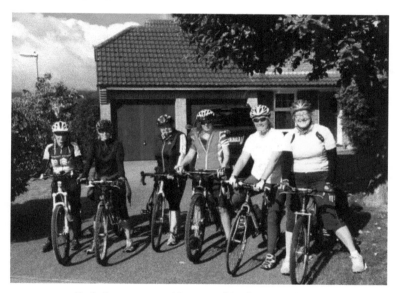

Brain trauma support team outside Liane's UK home

Since then, my doctor here in Australia has done a lot of research with colleagues worldwide and has found out that the inflammation of the brain was a rare side-effect of the arthritis drug that I had been taking. When I stopped taking medication, ready for the surgery, the body's immune system got rid of the symptoms.

Through all of that, the bike was my salvation. You can get on your bike and just enjoy nature. I ride a lot on my own but through my dark times I was supported on my rides by my friends from Breeze. When I came to Sydney, I was determined not to have a car and even more determined to explore the city by bike. I have done that, recovered and got to a place of better well-being.

Maybe there's something about women of a certain age who don't like being told, "You can't!"

I think, "I can!" And I do!

Liane Higham

CHAPTER 5

Snjezana Jojic

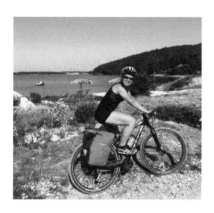

Snjezana left Bedfordshire to return to the rural village where she grew up in the Risnjak National Park near the Croatia - Slovenia border. Along with her partner, she's built a home from which she runs holidays, offering brown bear spotting, cycling, yoga and survival courses. In the UK, Snjezana lived in a concrete-covered area, but that didn't stop her from getting involved in cycling, quite the opposite!

SNJEZANA'S STORY

There's a lot of beautiful wildlife in Croatia. It's quiet with less traffic and less pollution. As I have got older, I have become aware of all those things. I left the UK because I wanted to get back to my roots and the natural surroundings that I grew up with. I think that being in the countryside can offer people something different, something important. I love taking people out into nature and showing them around so my partner and I have built a business in the village I grew up in so we can share the beauty of this place with others.

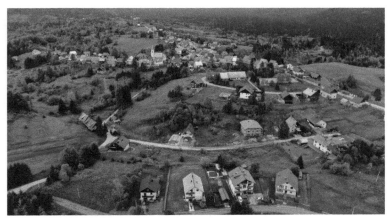

Panoramic view of Crni Lug where Snjezana runs her
holiday business offering brown bear spotting and cycling!

The brown bears live in Risnjak National Park alongside lynx and wolves. They don't obstruct people, only the farmers and there are very few of those in this area. The animals live deep in the forest so you won't come across one as a cyclist... unless you stay very still!

Getting fit is quite easy when I'm riding my bike in the mountains here... I don't have to go to the gym! When I go out of my house I can get straight on my bike and go up the road which is quiet too. I've got a circular route passing two lakes so I can stop at the lakes and have a swim. I am an adventurous person and I enjoy exploring.

For me, when I'm on a bike, it simplifies life, especially touring and all the things that I'd normally take for granted: a comfy bed, fireplace and showers. All that is gone. When you're touring, it's like your house is with you, on your bike. You cycle and you're surrounded by nature so nature is your new home. It's also freedom. Cycling gives you this feeling of complete freedom, the breeze that you feel and the satisfaction when you have completed something, a route or loop that you've planned.

On a long-distance tour, you get to know yourself better because you go through physical, emotional and mental hurdles. Sometimes you might think, "Oh God I'm never going to do this, I'm never going to get up that hill... Why did I do this in the first place?" These are all learning curves that teach you a lot about yourself.

When I planned a tour for other people, I discovered that it's even more challenging to manage others. Although I'd had experience working in sales, it was a different environment. When you've taken somebody away to a foreign country, it becomes a different scenario... Some people would not comply with what we asked them to do in terms of preparation. Sometimes that disrupted the dynamics of the team and it came down to me to manage the situation, to make it work without making anyone upset or angry.

We managed to help one lady all the way throughout the week and communicate with the other riders how they could also help her. She was struggling a lot, crying a lot and she wanted to quit but we all decided, "No, that's not why we are here, we not here to let people quit". It tested all my levels of communication, with the team, and then with the person that I was communicating the support to. It's not something you could learn from a textbook... We had to teach her about how to eat on a cycling holiday because she decided she was going to be on a diet. She had to climb hills and that was making her faint. We helped her and had to educate her whilst on the tour, which is all part of it. In some ways you have to expect anything and everything!

Our holidays in Croatia tend to be up to 50 miles a day with stops. Sometimes we do 40 miles over a full day. We stop for breaks in the morning, for lunch and then again in mid-afternoon. It's not about the speed, it's about somebody's mental state and head-space. I'm not a fast rider myself, I'm not competitive in that way. I like to enjoy the ride.

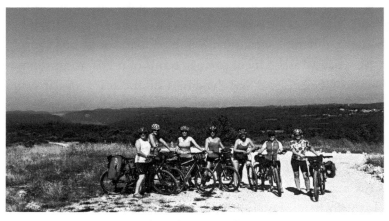

Croatian Adventure cycle tour

Touring in coastal Croatia, we eat a lot of fresh fish from the Adriatic when we are cycling. We also eat a lot of bananas and pick figs from the trees that we pass by on our bikes.

Nutrition is very important. I've learnt a lot about it over the years, mostly through personal experience. For instance, when I was cycle touring in colder countries such as Holland and the UK, it was important to keep my carbohydrates up and drink lots of water. I started every morning with porridge and filled up with pasta every evening. You've got to eat well to keep warm and keep going.

I've also done all sorts of jobs over the years. When I lived in the UK I had to do English courses to become an interpreter and then I did jobs in sales which improved my communication skills. Later, when I found out that there were jobs in cycle teaching, I jumped at the opportunity and worked on a number of initiatives at different organisations.

I've made some great friends through cycling. I met Liane Higham on a Breeze ride and we clicked instantly. I supported her Breeze rides and she supported mine. I also made friends with a girl called Sarah Maria who has got a website called, "Cycle Your Heart Out" and I visited her in Barcelona with another enthusiastic Breeze lady called Colette Holt to cycle a heart-shaped route! Again, Sarah Maria supported my Breeze rides. That was one of the amazing things about Breeze, it was all about supporting each other. To say "Thank you" I had a bear made, riding a bicycle!

If you are interested in a bespoke tour in the Croatian Mountains you can contact Snjezana via her website at www.pintarska.com. She offers accommodation and wildlife watching for up to six people.

When you're touring, it's like your house is with you, on your bike. You cycle and you're surrounded by nature so nature is your new home. It's freedom.

Snjezana Jojic

CHAPTER 6

Indigo Kelly-Forest

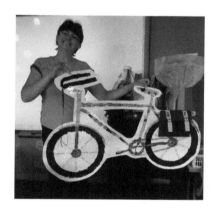

Indi was born in Bradford. She currently lives in rural Leicestershire surrounded by rolling countryside. Since starting bicycle touring, Indi's transformed from a size 24 woman who was too embarrassed to be seen on a bike to becoming a keen cyclist. As a ride leader, Indi guides from the back, allowing women to find their own pace and share their solutions. As the originator of many cycle touring adventures in France, Indi has been a great supporter of women in search of adventure. She has also featured on Cycling UK's list of 100 women in cycling.

INDI'S STORY

In 2009, I was a size 24 and my partner Al said we'd do the Bordeaux to Narbonne cycle ride along the Canal du Midi. "No! No! No!" I was terrified. Eventually she convinced me it would be okay. I said, "But I can't do 10 miles a day!" I was cross and bad tempered because I didn't want to do it.

We got to Bordeaux with loads of ridiculous kit, half of which we posted home after a few days. The first bit from Bordeaux to Creon, it's only twelve very gentle miles, but I can't tell you how many times we stopped because I couldn't cope.

I was struggling on the bike... Every hundred metres, I'd be stopping and out of breath. Every time there was shade, I'd stop to breathe and wonder, "What the...?"

As the trip went on, I started to become a little more confident and to see glimpses of the old me and, more importantly, new me. The only photograph at that time was me in profile, sitting cross-legged on the canal bank, wearing an enormous grey shirt and I was huge!

On the last few days of this journey of self-discovery, I managed a whopping 33 miles in one day. I was blown away! By the time we actually got towards the Mediterranean coast at Narbonne, I was going like the clappers. Al asked me what I had on my headphones and it was, "Bat Out of Hell." Al said, "That's exactly what you were doing!".

That 300 miles, from the beginning of that first tour to the end, changed me. They were massive changes but a lot of them were very subtle. It was only after the event that I started to think: "I've done this, so I could do that!"

And I did...

In 2012 I went on a course for Breeze Leadership Training with British Cycling and I'm still friends with the women who were on that course. I was so afraid of letting anyone down. All I could think was, "I can't lead women on rides!" I became an assistant leader for a while, until I could muster some confidence. Then, I started leading rides.

I was chatting to Susan Doram and some other friends and I told them about my 2009 adventure. They said, "Can you organise it for us?" I had the information and the route so I said "Yes!" That's how, in 2013, the "Women's French Adventures" began. It was terrifying. All those women! Suddenly I was advising women on cycle touring and camp craft! Fortunately, I was fast becoming a "nerd" in both areas!

The aim of the French Adventures was to have a positive impact on other women and pass on what Al had done for me. I remember one lady in particular. She came to meet me at a Breeze meeting up in the north-west with her two daughters who were in their late teens. They were all keen for her to go and do an adventure but she was so unsure about it. I managed to reassure her that I had been where she was now and to come along and join us.

On the day of the journey I had a call from the bus to say that she wasn't there at the meeting point. It turned out that her husband had tried to sabotage it but she had stood her ground and that was brilliant. Luckily the bus waited and she got on it.

That lady struggled throughout the whole of the trip. She was the first to wake up and last to leave... but she did it! I remember clearly that at the end of the trip, looking over at her when everyone was sitting chatting in a cafe. We were celebrating in the town square in the centre of Narbonne... And this woman, who had struggled throughout the trip, was sitting there so regally and she just had this confidence about her. I thought, "If I never do this again, she is my queen, she is the one I did it for." It sounds a bit grandiose but that's how I felt.

Since then, I have seen many women flourish - some almost imperceptibly and some voraciously; some in their "here and now" and some "after the fact."

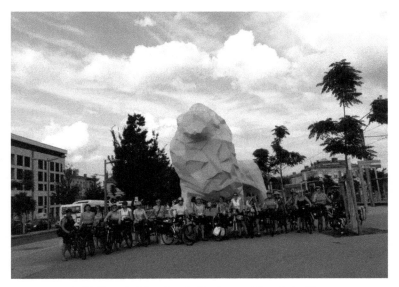

Indi's French Adventure in Bordeaux at the start of Les Deux Mers

Little did I know on that first French Adventure in 2013 that I was becoming ill. I didn't have any money so I was living on scraps. I took high-sugar caffeine powders with me from the UK so I had energy to cycle. I was living on those and they were compounding the problem. It was just a survival strategy. I started to get much slimmer. I was craving sugar, the one thing I shouldn't have been having, and I didn't realise I was dropping more and more weight. I was doing more exercise but I didn't know anything about diabetes.

At a Doctor's appointment, I discovered that blood sugars are supposed to be between four and seven. Mine were 34, which I now know is frightening and could have put me in to a coma. I continued to lose weight and size 8 hung off me. I was a size six and, in the bath, I had to have a very thick cushion because my bones hurt. I ended up having to have a couple of toppers on the mattress because the little buttons would hurt. I had neuropathy in my legs. My nerve endings were damaged and would never fully recover. I had two metal frames on the bed to hold the duvet off my skin. I slept in a tunnel for a long time.

When I was first diagnosed in 2014, the diabetes nurses said that I must not get on my bike for at least three months. I was an emotional wreck anyway. I had to take Metformin and Gliclazide tablets every day. They just made me feel sick. I went on various courses with the diabetes nurses that started to explain things to me and I remember asking, "When will I be able to stop all this?" They said, "This is it for the rest of your life," and of course I had a meltdown. It took several years to get up to a size 10 and feel comfortable and even then, I was still an emotional wreck. By then, I was able to cycle again.

The few times I began to cycle, I had to learn to balance between exercise and taking insulin because if you do both you could end up in a coma. There were several times where I'd have to pull over to the side of the road to have a sugar-laden cereal bar and I got to the point where I could smell sugar which made me feel sick but I'd have to eat it. Cyclists would pull over and ask if I was OK. They would chat to me for 10-15 minutes and make sure I was okay and they would talk about their mates who have diabetes. It became normalised and that was amazing.

During these very difficult Covid-19 times, cycling has once again helped me to maintain some kind of emotional and physical equilibrium. I've pedalled many "socially distanced" miles alone, yet not alone. I always call out "Hello!" and "Isn't it lovely to be out?" to anyone I see and everyone, without exception, has responded wonderfully. Thank you! It really does make my day when people say, "Hi!"

Within and beyond these adventures, I've met and grown in the company of so many inspirational and wonderful women. I feel truly blessed. I wish I could name each and everyone of them. I hope from my heart that you each know who you are!

That first tour changed me. They were massive changes but a lot of them were very subtle. It was only after the event that I started to think, "I've done this... so I could do that!"

Indigo Kelly-Forest

CHAPTER 7

Sarah Layden

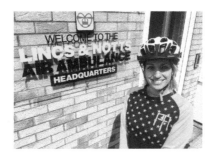

Sarah is a community nurse in Carlton, Nottinghamshire. She is softly spoken and, at first, a little bit shy... but beneath that calm exterior, she's a mountain-biking addict, flying through the air in the woods at every opportunity! It's a risky business but Sarah loves it. She has an incredible survival story and now she's a brand ambassador and fund-raiser. Riding her bike is something which makes her feel very much alive. When I asked her if it was pure adrenaline, she admitted, "Probably...but I do like all forms of cycling, from full-suspension mountain bikes to e-bikes".

SARAH'S STORY

In my early twenties I was living on my own so joining cycling clubs and mountain biking was a great way of meeting people and sharing what I enjoyed. I soon got hooked and was riding two or three nights a week. I met my partner and, with encouragement from him, I got a better bike.

Everything was going well. I was about to start a new position as a Health Visitor and I had some time off. I hadn't planned on riding the day of my accident but I ended up joining my partner and some friends who were already out riding in Bestwood Country Park.

In mountain biking there are things that you should never say and never do. "That one last run"... that one last run that's hard to resist, even when you're tired. My partner Ryan warned me, "You probably shouldn't do it." But I wanted to do it. He got his phone out to film me.

I was cycling down a technical route in a quarry with a vertical drop-off. I clipped my front wheel and cartwheeled over my handlebars off my bike. I can't remember what happened next but I know that I fell thirty feet and landed on my head.

Ryan thought I was dead. He threw his phone down to run to me and then didn't have a phone to call the emergency services.

Ryan called over to my friend, "We're going to need to call the Air Ambulance". It was quite closed off where we were, there was no road access. If I hadn't had the Air Ambulance, I would have died. They got me to Intensive Care in three minutes.

On the impact, my brain shot forwards and backwards, making it swell. Later I had to have a bolt in my head to let the pressure out. The staff at A&E took Ryan and my parents into the room of doom. The surgeons had to prepare everyone and say, "She's going into surgery and she might not make it."

Luckily, I surprised everyone.

I only spent four weeks in hospital then I went to Linden Lodge where the Traumatic Brain Injury (TBI) team worked hard to rehabilitate me. My mum told me to never ride a bike again, but in rehab, the first thing I did was get on to a static bike.

Perhaps fortunately, I didn't have any memory when I woke up. I didn't know that I'd had an accident on my bike, I thought I'd been in a car accident. I'd only got happy memories of cycling and I wanted to get on that static bike to get some exercise.

I don't know if the fitness from the cycling helped with my recovery... It probably did. I had a lot of fatigue, which I still suffer from now, and I couldn't ride my bike straight away. I suffered with memory problems and the TBI team came to see me regularly at home.

The specialists didn't think I would get back to work but I managed. I'm working part-time now because of the fatigue. It's been hard but I think you've got to fight. I'm a bit more careful now, more cautious, but I still like cycling. Actually, I LOVE it!

I've got all sorts of bikes now, including an e-bike which I won because of my story. I wasn't too sure at first, but I find it amazing and it means that I can cycle further. With my e-bike, I don't have to take my car to places, I can cycle there and cycle home and do more miles.

I love travelling to take part in downhill adventures and I've been to the States and Morzine in the French Alps since the accident. I had to take a normal bike abroad because you can't fly with the e-bike batteries.

My mum is not too pleased, but I tell her it's safe. Actually, since the Covid-19 lockdown, I've converted both my mum and dad to cycling which is a big achievement for all of us!

After my accident and recovery. I met up with the Air Ambulance crew to say an enormous "Thank You". If I had gone by road to hospital, I wouldn't have made it. Now I fund-raise for them. I can't thank them enough.

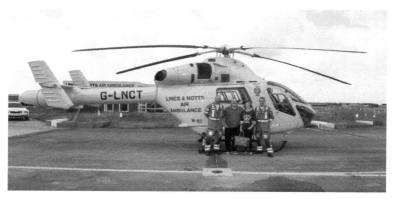

Lincs and Notts Air Ambulance

I've got all sorts of bikes now including an e-bike. I wasn't too sure at first but I find it amazing and it means that I can cycle further.

Sarah Layden

CHAPTER 8

Ruth McIntosh

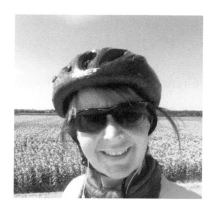

Ruth lives on the edge of Sheffield in a village in north-east Derbyshire. She didn't choose to be a cycle ride leader for Breeze because she was confident, she did it to commit time to cycling. Her life wasn't very adventurous at that point, with the responsibilities of being a forty-something mum, teacher and wife being very demanding of her time and energy. Fortunately, she was about to rediscover herself and find a new sense of freedom.

RUTH'S STORY

British Cycling's Breeze initiative got women to do things together that we didn't yet have the confidence or strength to do on our own. I loved being a volunteer leader. Women would turn up with all the gear looking for moral support to get started. That was the point of Breeze: to allow women to cycle in a supportive and friendly environment where they could enjoy riding traffic-free routes at their own pace.

Enter Super-Gran, a woman in the group, "My dad never let me get on a bike as a kid, because I was a girl, but it's something I've always wanted to do." She then needed a quick "m" check on her shiny white bike and her helmet altered before I could give her a "crash" course in cycling. Fortunately, she was amazing and had a broad smile that lit up her face when she cycled. She gripped on to that bike for dear life and gave it her all, spinning like mad. A life-long ambition realised, Super-Gran was completely elated!

After leading rides for a year, I decided to strike out on my own to see if I could go further afield. It was hard to get started at times but as soon as I got on the bicycle, I was drifting away along the country lanes. Cycling was a great escape. At work my teaching methods were being questioned and my workload was being increased. In truth, we were all being squeezed but it felt very stressful because I was already working at full-tilt. At the same time, my marriage was ending, after nearly twenty years of us being together. My home life and work life were both in tatters.

Throughout this difficult period, my parents, my sister Ellen and cycling kept me going. Then, one day, whilst scrolling through Facebook, an image of sunflowers burst in to my brain and lifted my heart. It was an advert aimed at the Breeze community for a women-only week-long bicycle tour along Le Canal du Midi in France in the summer holidays. "That's it! I'm going! Woohoo! Troubles be gone!"

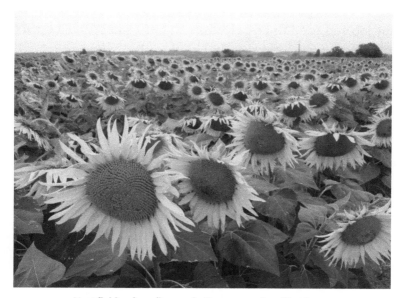

Vast fields of sunflowers in France... and smiling faces everywhere!

I knew I could cycle a reasonable distance on the flat and I was longing to be somewhere new. The idea of rolling along canal tow paths and country lanes surrounded by new experiences and nature really appealed to me. Plus, it would be all women so there would always be someone available to help!

The woman leading the French Adventure was Indigo Kelly-Forest, or Indi as I came to know her. I thought she'd be dead posh but she was a down-to-earth northerner with an infectious laugh and wicked sense of humour. I first met her when she hosted a pre-trip get together at her house, to practise putting up our tents and talk about bike camping kit. I was a bit of a mess that first night: tired, confused, grumbling about my job and soon-to-be-ex husband... but I soon perked up after a glass of wine and a giggle with the other women.

Indi said, "This is going to be a great journey for you," hinting at the holiday being a transformational experience in the spiritual sense. Inwardly, I scoffed a little, "I'm just riding my bike across France."

In fact, the holiday brought about a big shift in my attitude. I was determined to navigate my own way, to ride at my own pace and enjoy the sheer freedom of a full week freewheeling through the most glorious scenery. It was a totally liberating feeling, to be able to head in one direction and actually get somewhere with only my own luggage and thoughts.

At times it was physically demanding but it was also ridiculously good fun.

I found myself being able to laugh again! The whole experience gave me the strength I needed to manage and take control of my life. Crucially, I reverted back to my maiden name, regained my identity and started to recover from the heart-break. I found some wonderful things to love: good company, great food and cycling!

The other thing I fell in love with, and this surprised me a little, was France. I had always wanted to speak another language fluently and struggled like mad with languages when I was younger. That year in France, I was overwhelmed by the friendliness of the French people I met along the Canal du Midi. I even managed to understand what was being said and speak a word or two of French myself.

With time to notice things around me, all my senses were heightened to absorb the sounds, colours, tastes and reflections. There was an immense beauty in the scale of the landscape, tall sunflowers as big as my head, big skies, long baguettes. It put my problems into perspective. The days were long but I always made it with time to rebuild my house, also known as "the tent" and I slept well.

I got lost just once, where the canal split in two and I had to choose which prong of the fork pointed the way. It was the longest day, three days in to the trip and I was stretched to my limit. I had decided to travel totally alone that day so I was forced into having my wits about me and observing markers in the landscape.

Luckily, I got a really strange feeling... A hundred metres down the track, all my senses were on full alert. It felt wrong: the bustling path that I had been following seemed quiet and under-used. Out of nowhere, a French farmer appeared carrying a shotgun and surrounded by barking dogs. "Turn back! Turn back!" I spoke aloud to myself and turned around whilst thinking, "Thank God I was mindful enough to notice those signs!"

Not immediately after that trip, but a few years later, I conceded with a smile that Indi had been right. Giving myself a week once a year is an incredible freedom and it gives me the space I need to re-examine myself and change the way I think. Whilst my future may be uncertain, I'm more flexible and re-silient. I *can* make new friends, find a new job, discover new hobbies. I can change and face the future with hope.

Now my children are old enough to start experiencing adventures for themselves and I look back on my journey surprised at how far I've come. Whilst I got in to Breeze to help others, being part of something bigger has helped me enormously and this book is a tribute to the power of a great initiative.

I've got an extra hobby now, "blogging" about experiential slow travelling for fun at www.slow-cycle.com (because I'm a slow-plodder of a cyclist!) Day-dreaming about sunflowers keeps me going through dark cold winters. I also love supporting people and working collaboratively on writing projects. Writing about the experiences of others helps me to discover new places and make new connections... sowing the seeds for stories yet to come.

There was an immense beauty in the scale of the landscape...

It put my problems into perspective.

Ruth McIntosh

CHAPTER 9

Janet Steel

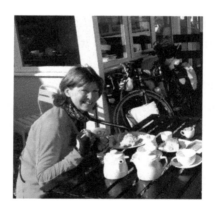

Steel by name, steel by nature! Janet is an experienced cyclist so it's a surprise to learn that she didn't learn to cycle as a child; her parents denied her access to a bike by saying that she had no road sense! Learning to ride in her 20s, for many years she only used her bike for commuting. Later, when she reached semi-retirement, Janet learned how to cycle effectively and she claims that she's still honing her technique. She doesn't get older, she just gets better. Read on to find out how she pedals to test her mettle.

JANET'S STORY

My parents let my older brother cycle and they always said, "Janet can't go on the bike because she's got no road sense," so I got cut off from getting on the bike. I didn't even get on my brother's bike because he used to disappear on adventures to a reservoir. I didn't even see him on it.

My husband taught me to cycle. One of the first things we did was to cycle to see our friends and stay overnight. And then we never did anymore. Later, when we moved to Bromsgrove in our late twenties, I used to cycle nine miles to work.

About twenty years ago, when I went into early semi-retirement, I got an allotment. A guy came over to me one day and said, "You like cycling and walking, don't you?" I said, "Yes."

He said, "My wife is looking for someone to cycle with." We met up and started doing little bike rides. She knew people who had done touring on bikes following CTC and Sustrans route so she and I started doing the same. We chose 100 mile routes and we'd do about 30 miles a day for three and a half days then get the train back. We called ourselves, "The Cycling

Gardeners" because we'd got into it from being on the allotment.

We made loads of mistakes. We did no training! I carried loads of clothes but didn't have any protective cycling shorts. I didn't know anything about cycling properly or how to change gears and my cog came off all the time. On the first trip, I took a heavy book with me and we stayed in Bed & Breakfasts so it was more upmarket than the cycle camping I do now.

After a year or so I saw an advert at the local swimming pool and it was a woman advertising a cycling club. This would be about the year 2000. I got in touch with her and she was a very inspirational woman. She had been out with a cycling group of speedy cyclists and they dropped her and her mate. It was mostly chaps at that time and this woman and her friend had to make their own way home. They hadn't prepped the route and they didn't know where they were. That experience really annoyed her so she said, "I'm going to start my own group and it's not going to be like that." It was going to have a completely different ethos, "We won't ever drop anybody, we're not going to have different grades of cycling within the group, we'll go with the slowest cyclist and encourage people from the back." If you wanted to start cycling faster, it would be time for you to find a "sporty" club. She still runs a group along those lines. She taught me everything I know about cycling although I started out by just getting on the bike. My son says there's a difference between people who ride bikes and cyclists and I can see where he's coming from.

I've cycled in various places, around the Golden Ring in Russia starting and ending in Moscow, the Camino de Santiago, the Scotland 500, France and in the UK. I don't think much about the cycling when I'm on the bike but beforehand I set targets, realistic targets. I know I'm ageing and cycling with people quite a bit younger than me. The group I'm in now has got chaps in it as well but they're good chaps and they never leave anybody behind. They're the strongest so they go at the back to get people out of trouble if they need to, the strongest doesn't go at the front. Nevertheless, I like to set targets.

I suffer a lot with saddle sores so I phoned a friend and said, "If you were me and he wanted to get fit what would you do in the shortest amount of time, would you do hills or distance?" He responded, "I'd do hills, every time."

I thought I'd take that bit of advice and I found a hill that starts about four miles away. I decided to go up and down the hill as many times as I could until it was time to go home. The hill has got five different roads up and down it so I varied the route to keep my strength up and build my legs. I suppose I enjoy gaining that physical strength.

For me, a hill is a driver. Often you can't start your bike on a hill because you're in too low a gear to get any pressure. My attitude is: I'd rather kill myself to get to the top of the hill than stop and not be able to get on the bike again. It's not so I can say, "I've got to the top of the hill," it's just easier than stopping and trying to get back on the bike. I think, "I can count to ten pedal strokes to get to the top of that"... and then it won't be enough so I'll do more!

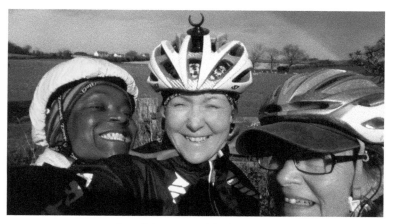

From left, Susan, Nicky and Janet

I don't think much about the cycling when I'm on the bike but beforehand I set targets, realistic targets.

Janet Steel

CHAPTER 10

Janine Morrall

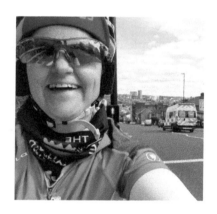

Teeny Janine is based in North Sheffield, Hillsborough. Sheffield is bloody hilly so she must be a bit bonkers to start cycling through commuting, especially as she lives on the top of the hill so the only downhill is towards town and then you've got to get back up! A nanny by day, Janine has a talent for engaging people in activity making her a natural Breeze Leader, Cycle trainer and advocate for participation in cycling. Give her a wave if you see her cycling around Sheffield. Janine's the tiny one with a smile on her face and a shock of colour in her hair.

JANINE'S STORY

I moved back to Sheffield in 2008. Some of my friends had just trained as spinning instructors, so I was supporting them by going to their classes. When I met my now husband in 2010, he questioned me, "If you sit in a gym on a bike, why don't you cycle?" We bought a couple of cheap bikes in early 2011 and started to commute to work on them.

Cycling was a way of getting around without having to spend money. It meant not sitting on the tram, catching everyone's germs. Then it really grew on me when the Olympics happened and the Tour de France came to the north of Sheffield. We got caught up in all that excitement. I rang British Cycling to ask if they were doing a Sky Ride in Sheffield and that's when they suggested Breeze to me. I said, "I've never led a ride or done group leading". They said, "It doesn't matter, we're not looking for experienced cyclist group riders, we've been there and done that".

The best thing about Breeze is working with women who aren't really sure why they bought a bike or got it out of the shed. After a couple of rides, they've gone on from doing one lap of Dam Flask reservoir to two or maybe a 20 miler. Seeing them make progress and achieve something is great, it doesn't have to be a World Record or anything. We get a lot of people who come on their own, then they'll bring their friends afterwards. I get some ladies returning a couple of times then I don't see them again. I always wonder: are they still cycling?

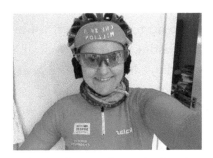

**Janine is a long-serving cycle champion
based in Sheffield**

There are some people who live in cities who might be put off cycling by the lack of infrastructure. A lot of consultation needs to be done with communities and businesses. How do we involve the whole community, even if people don't necessarily want to cycle themselves? There's a lot of information that people probably don't realise even exists; you don't see it unless you walk or use public transport. Since Paralympian Dame Sarah Storey started as a Travel Ambassador in Sheffield, there has been more investment and they've started to join up the dots that were dead ends before. Hopefully, we're making progress.

A group of four of us tour in the UK. We decide on a route, book the days off work and off we go, sharing accommodation along the way. Touring takes time. You'll see a sign that says, "1 mile" to somewhere then see another four blue and white Sustrans signs over the next 5 miles saying the same thing! You're always having to phone the B&B to say, "We'll get there when we get there, sorry." For day trips we head east where it is flatter than Sheffield! We tend to do northern routes for our longer tours so Coast and Castles, Hadrian's Wall and The Way of the Roses, gradually working around remote parts.

I've not got the greatest balance in the world and I've had surgery on my ears over the years. I don't like labels but I'm probably slightly dyspraxic. I was about nine or ten before I was able to tie my shoelaces. I've never been good at ball sports and I've struggled with coordination. In dance classes everybody would be going to the left with their right leg in the air and I'd be going to the right with my left leg in the air!

Recently I took part in a study where they put me on the Watt bike and fitted me with brainwave sensors. The area of the brain that usually lights up when you're riding a bike didn't, instead another area did to compensate for it. Their conclusion was that I probably shouldn't be able to ride but I can! I always laughed off stuff that I don't find easy and got on with it.

I say to people, "I'm not bothered what bike you come on because, actually, it's you that's powering the bike." It's about your physical and mental determination not the five-grand bike. You can have a really expensive bike and not do anything with it or you could have a bike that's £100 that you bought from your friend and if you're determined to get up Winnat's Pass, a very steep incline, you're going to get up it!

I'm not bothered what bike you cycle on because it's you that's powering the bike. It's about your physical and mental determination.

Janine Morrall

CHAPTER 11

Joanne Westwood

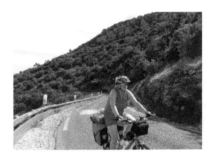

Joanne is made from Lancashire grit: strong stuff! Although she always seems like one of the most relaxed riders in a group, underneath she's surprisingly stubborn and determined. She's also quick to learn from all those veterans who hammer out the miles with a youthful zeal. Honestly, it's not all uphill for Joanne because she secretly loves to attack a gradient so that she can look back on her achievement and feel a glow instead of a burn!

JOANNE'S STORY

I have a big picture of Mont Ventoux on my kitchen wall that I carted around France on my bike rack-pack for a week after I cycled up it. Susan Doram and I went into this little bric-a-brac shop and we found these repro posters from the 50s. It's a very cool image showing Mont Ventoux and there's some text written in French... *"you must zee zis beautiful place before you leave Provence."*

I look at that picture and I think: "I can probably do just about anything now," because there was no way I thought I could cycle up that... and I did! It took me hours! Kids were passing me on bikes that were too small and they were wearing sandals...

"Urgh!" I was crying. "STOP IT!" Beforehand I was thinking, "I'll stop about every four or 5K" and I was stopping about every 500m at some points. It was really hard. I didn't push, I cycled, but it was really steep in places and I was barely moving anywhere up the hill! Ventoux wasn't on my bucket list as such but... *"When you're going to that part of France, you should do it."* There was no question about it: I was going to do it so I did!

It was the same the first year I went touring. I was going to do it, no matter how hard it was. And it it was hard and really hot. All of the others were really tough resilient women, especially the older ones that had done it before or had more cycling experience. They just absolutely hammered it. It was really good being around women like that because I learned about touring from them. They had lightweight tents and mine weighed a tonne!

I thought, why has everyone got a Kindle? Why didn't you bring books like me? I had taken big thick books to cart around on the bike for hundreds of miles and a huge towel. Not like a little handy towel: a stupid bath towel. Somebody went home on the first trip and they lived near to where I had parked my car so I said, "Can you take these back?" They took the towel and a load of books. That was about 5kg of weight gone. I didn't realise that weight was really important when I first started! I didn't really know much about bikes! I liked having a bike. I'd had a bike as a kid and I used to go to work on my bike... Until I didn't. As an adult, I didn't really know about bikes as a form of transport or adventure. Funnily enough, I did as a kid but I'd forgotten that.

I used to cycle with my sister and we'd go to this place near to where we used to live in Blackpool. It wasn't very far from home and we called it "Past Warreners" which was a Cash and Carry on a big industrial estate. My mum would say, "Where have you been?" And we'd say, "Past Warreners", so she'd say,

"Well, don't go any further than that." We were on elastic and our boundaries only stretched so far. We could go to the beach alone but we could only paddle in the sea.

I like the absurdity of cycling and stumbling on unusual places. Once I was having a tough day, having not slept. My eyes were all swollen from sleeping in a tent and I looked like I'd been crying all night. This didn't deter an over-friendly Frenchman who wanted me to go back to his house. I missed the turning for the campsite somewhere outside Toulouse because I was pedalling like a mad woman to escape. I didn't want to look over my shoulder and encourage him. I was lost, disorientated and desperate for the toilet. There was a short path that led to a Wild-West themed hotel in the middle of nowhere. It was really busy with diners. I thought, "What the bloody hell is this?" I was sweaty, grimy and minging, so I just snuck in and used the loo. What else could I do? Now, of course, it's funny and a highlight of my trip. I get a strange buzz when things go wrong!

I had first found Breeze as a participant. I liked the idea of cycling with women in a group and the Breeze leaders were really funny, really comical with proper banter all the time so you were having a laugh as well as chatting to other women. When I think back now, we just used to go up and down the docks for three miles for an hour and a half or something and had lots of stops. I did the training and the First-aid course and started doing rides as a leader.

Breeze was good because women made the time to do it. I used to put rides on a Saturday or Sunday afternoon and I'd think, "I bet some of these poor buggers have had to cook a Sunday dinner before they come out for a bike ride!" I think it's really interesting that the bicycle was part of the suffragette movement. It was an important way of women getting freedom and the suffragettes had special outfits to cycle in. I didn't know until I did Breeze that in some cultures it's not really seen as an appropriate pastime for a woman. I think that's bonkers really because it's a way of getting around as much as it is something that we use for leisure. Sometimes, in my headier moments I think, "I'm just going to get rid of my car and ride my bike all the time."

I like a good country route with that sense of discovery. There are some hills near me in the Trough of Bowland and my eldest son used to live in Lancaster when he was at university. I'd drive home on this back road and I thought, "I could cycle, this isn't that far", in a car of course, speeding along! So I did it... On a horrendously heavy metal mountain bike. It was too hard... I launched the bike in to the bushes when I got to the top and bawled my eyes out!

Eventually I realised that I needed to get back on my bike, "Go home you idiot! Get on with it: nobody is going to come and rescue you!" At the time I needed to physically challenge myself. And it did really challenge me!

Afterwards I thought, "Well, I did that, so I know I can do it!" People used to say, "If you cycle, you'll get the miles in your legs," and that's what I felt. Cycling makes that happen immediately: you get that impact of your success in being able to climb a mountain or cycle really fast for five seconds. You get instant gratification from it, especially in beautiful locations in France or the UK. There's nothing better than being on your bike!

I am fitter now than when I started cycling. The discipline of cycling, planning, eating properly and resting helped me to develop a healthier lifestyle. I am a work in progress!

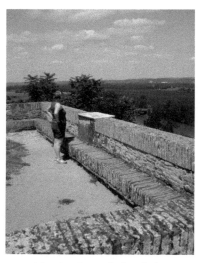

The view is worth the climb!

At the time I needed to physically challenge myself.

And cycling did really challenge me.

Joanne Westwood

CHAPTER 12

Nicky Woods

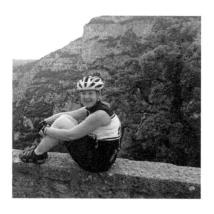

Like many of us, Nicky has found cycling to be a great way to deal with the stress of a difficult job in sales with crazy hours. She started cycling seriously by getting into Mountain Biking, which is not for the faint-hearted and it gave her an exciting taste of the great outdoors. After getting into cycling, she then discovered touring and camping. She loves all the gear and she's a self-professed gadget-queen! In recent years she's moved from Mansfield near Nottingham to the Scottish Borders and taken the gear to the extreme by buying a large motorhome with all mod cons.

NICKY'S STORY

I was a Forces child and we moved a lot. The first bike I remember riding was in America. It was a proper pretty girls' bike, all pink, white and chrome with a flowery basket on the front. We brought the bike back to the UK with us. I've always been really clumsy and I remember cycling down some steps at the end of a cul-de-sac. I cut my hand along the side of the handlebars before I fell off and ripped the flesh on my hand wide open. I've still got a scar.

I got into biking properly when I lived in Mansfield about eleven years ago. A friend gave me an unwanted bike. It was an Apollo from Halfords. I thought, "Right! I'm going to get fit!" and I cycled three miles to my friend Tanya's house. I was knackered! Tanya put the bike in the back of her car and took me home and the bike sat at home, unloved, for ages. I started cycling occasionally around Sherwood Pines and I got the biking bug! To be honest, I didn't know how to ride a bike properly. I even buckled the back wheel of that bike. I knew nothing about bikes.

I bought myself a half-decent Mountain Bike but it was still quite heavy. I gradually kept upgrading as I learnt new bike skills. My local mountain-biking trail centre had graded routes so I started doing the "easy" green route which is about six miles long. I was exhausted! Eventually, I was doing the more challenging red route and I got faster. I met a lady called Dee who was working on the Breeze initiative. She taught me a lot. Prior to this, I had been falling off just about every ride. I was always organising rides so Dee suggested that I become a Breeze champ. I also did a bit of leading for Sherwood Pines Cycling Club.

I met Indi and Susan when they came to a Breeze meeting. They talked about the Women's French Adventure and I went along in the second year, 2014. That's when I got really into touring. The French Adventure was tough at times. By the fifth day I was feeling a bit run down and exhausted. Touring is different because you are on your bike day after day so it's a shock to the system.

The next morning, I was about to set off with a couple of ladies when one of the ladies said, "We're going to start with a bit of a hill." I had a meltdown and burst into tears. Indi saw this, swooped me up out of the situation and put things in to perspective for me. Indi said, "You CAN do this!" We had done 80 miles the day before, whilst other people had done 50, and it was hot. I said, "Okay: I CAN do this!" and I plodded up *that* hill. Every time I come to a difficult hill now, I always remember that hill and I think, "This might be tough but it won't beat me." I know I can do difficult stuff and that gives me confidence.

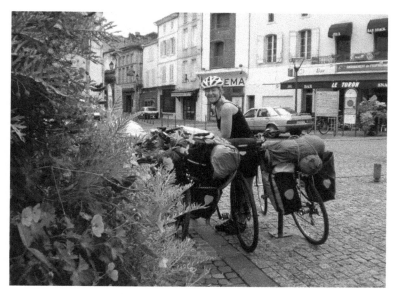

Nicky sorting out her gear in France

Cycling and dog walks have always been my stress busters. They're therapeutic. As a single parent I've always had to work hard to make ends meet and always had to take better paid, more stressful jobs. I managed for a while then there was a problem which put me in a dark place. At the same time I lost my dog Bessie to cancer.

I was an area manager and the job had become increasingly demanding on my time. Previously, I'd managed to get home on a Tuesday or Thursday night which were girls' cycling nights. That was my way of keeping stress levels low. Then, the more corporate I got, the less time I had out on my bike... And the more the stress levels got the better of me. I needed the endorphins I get from exercise to get my heart rate up and feel alive.

I continued working silly hours and stress got the better of me. When mum moved to Scotland, I'd go to visit her at weekends. My heart would lift with joy when I saw the "Scotland" sign. There was no phone signal after I had left the motorway, so no one could contact me and that gave me a wave of relief and euphoria. Then there would be six miles of beautiful countryside and I knew that I could relax and breathe. I decided to sell up, leave work and move to Scotland.

I now live in Scotland alongside my mum with a motorhome, kit store and collection of bikes. I love Scotland, the scenery, the people and the tranquility. I've got a new plan and I'm going to retrain so I can make better choices about how I earn a living. I've been on a long journey to get here and the cycling has helped with that. The biggest thing I like about biking is the companionship. I like my own company but now I'm better at saying, "Yes, let's go and do this!" Since that first trip with the WFA, I've organised lots of other trips and done one or two big challenges every year. I've cycled in northern Spain on the route of The Camino de Santiago on my own, done a coast to coast in a day for charity and cycled up Mont Ventoux on a hybrid.

When the Covid crisis is over, I'm hoping to do more in the tourist industry in Scotland and I'll be using my motorhome and bike more. I've now got the confidence I need to find a rural spot and park up in the middle of nowhere with no one around, just me and my dog.

Every time I come to a hill I think, this is going to take a lot of energy but I'm going to keep going. I know I can do difficult stuff and that gives me confidence.

Nicky Woods

Riding your bike: lessons learned

After interviewing all of the wonderful women who contributed their stories to this book in lockdown, I felt a lot of enthusiasm for the future and got the sense that maybe my best cycling years were still yet to come... This is what I learned:

1. You don't get older, you get wiser!

2. Sh*t happens... you'll deal with it.

3. A week of cycling is a year's worth of adventure.

4. Cycling in a group keeps you going, you'll take it in turns to laugh or cry!

5. Strangers are kind to cyclists, because they think you're bonkers!

6. Life is beautiful when you're travelling at 7-15 mph.

7. When you're cycling, food is fuel, and everything tastes better after a pedal.

8. Hills can bring out strong emotions.

9. Riding in circles is OK. Over time, the circles might get bigger

10. Screaming at goats is more fun than lying on a beach!

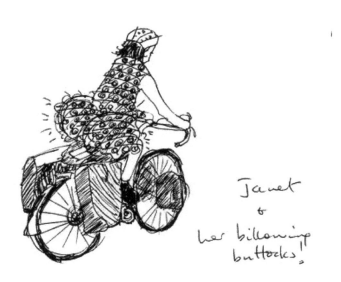

Janet
to
her billowing
buttocks!

Illustration by Dorothy Craw

Choosing a bike

Contrary to popular belief, riding a bike doesn't have to be a strenuous or uncomfortable activity. In fact, riding a bicycle is five times more energy efficient than walking. For touring and traffic-free cycling, your bike should be sturdy enough for gravel paths but light and smooth enough to make pedalling fun. It doesn't really matter if you ride a sit up and beg or road bike with drops, as long as you are comfortable.

Mountain Bikes

I had a mountain bike with front suspension for years, which was comfortable but heavy. Full suspension, involving bouncy forks or moving parts which smooth out the ride, is essentially designed for downhill comfort and absorbing shocks, which adds weight to the bike. Mountain bike tyres are usually wide and knobbly to grip on to loose gravel surfaces, ideal for off-roading and dirt trails. Changing to smoother tyres will make cycling on beaten-flat gravel trails easier.

Hybrids

My current bike is a mid-range hybrid. A hybrid or everyday bike has a strong frame, robust tyres, smooth gears, flat or riser handlebars and the facility to attach a rack for luggage. With a cross between the speed of a road bike and the gearing of a mountain bike, hybrids are lightweight but sturdy. The upright riding position also makes them ideal for cycling in traffic and commuting through town so they're a good everyday option.

Gravel Bikes

Gravel bikes are a new breed of bikes that have become popular in recent years. These look more like road bikes but they have been subtly adapted for all terrains by the addition of specialist tyres and gears. Gravel bikes tend to appeal to road bike users who are looking to explore rougher off-road terrain. Experienced cyclists are also now turning to more lightweight bike-packing on their tours, buying specially made bags to fit their frames.

Road Bikes

Road bikes are lightweight bikes with smooth thin tyres. They usually have drop handlebars and they are built for road riding at speed. Generally the older the rider, the better the road bike!

Folding Bikes

Traditionally these are commuter or city bikes with a folding frame, tall seat stem and small wheels. Some people choose to tour on these because they are portable and have an upright position allowing you to look around and enjoy the scenery.

Tyres

The quickest of all fixes is to inflate the tyres fully so you can't pinch them. If this doesn't work, it's worth getting new inner tubes rather than attempting a repair, especially as you can now buy puncture resistant inner tubes. To go a step further, buy smoother puncture-resistant tyres. Replacing knobbly MTB tyres with slicks or hybrid tyres will make a difference to your efficiency on Sustrans trails, although they're not quite as good on loose gravel.

Gears

Ideally you need enough gears to avoid grinding so you can pedal at a comfortable gear. The number of gears you will need will depend on where you live or where you want to tour. Most modern bikes have enough gears, 18 or 21.

Saddle

You need your hips and seat (bum) to stay level when you are cycling. And do stay seated for goodness sake! Touring for most of the day is nothing like spinning in the gym so you need to pace yourself. For a while I had my seat too high; too low is more common for beginners. Basically, you need your leg to be slightly bent when the pedal is at its lowest point.

Weight and Cost

A touring bike could weigh 17-18kg if you include pedals, a comfortable saddle, bottle cages and rear luggage rack. My Specialized Touring bike weighs 18kg and cost £500 in a sale. Weights vary from 14kg - 20kg. Over 20 kg might be too heavy as you're going to be carrying 10-15 kg of extra weight if you're camping. Plus, if you're like me, there might be a bit extra on your body! A light road bike might be only 7-8 kg but won't be as comfortable on trails.

Still Unsure?

Don't let fretting over these details stop you and don't be afraid to ask for help. You can always upgrade as you go. A good bike shop will help you and there are loads of women friendly cycling forums where you can ask for advice. The important thing is to get started. When I'm in France or National Parks in the UK, I rent bikes and they're about the same quality as my hybrid in the UK. Try to avoid trends and stick to your criteria!

E-Bikes

E-bikes are fantastic and perfect for getting back into shape, going up hills and mid-distance touring. They're also pricey and you get what you pay for. Although e-biking has taken off in the UK, it's much more acceptable in other European countries where there's less bike snobbery and more understanding of using bikes as transport. Two of the women in this book use e-bikes for transport instead of driving cars and a third uses an e-bike regularly for leisure.

Using an e-bike is NOT cheating as they only offer assistance through cadence sensors. The harder you're pushing the more they kick in.

Before you invest in electric, do your research. Bike hire can be excellent value and there's no better way of getting a feel for the level of assistance, weight or noise they make before you buy. Some are very quiet and they're great to ride. Be careful, they're addictive!

Mileage planning for cycle touring

Daily mileage can be anything you want. Moderately mobile beginners will be able to manage 25 miles to 50 miles a day. In kilometres this will be 40-80 km, impressively more! Remember, you can take all day and you are on your own journey.

For me slow living is good living. A ride can feel like a whole weekend away and a tour makes me feel like I have gone back in time and turned back the clock.

Cycling traffic-free (in any country) is not like cycling in your local town or city. Once you get your balance the pace is up to you. Just keep moving at a pace which you feel comfortable with.

Rough guidance on daily mileage/levels:

1. Easy: 10-20 miles on flat terrain
2. Gentle: 15-30 miles on flat terrain with some undulations

3. Moderate: 20-45 miles on gravel tracks with some climbs
4. Active: 30-50 miles on uneven ground with climbs
5. Challenging: 50-80 miles on loose ground and challenging terrain

Some of these distances might seem nothing to a road cyclist but when you're on a traffic-free gravel path progress is slower and you'll feel all the lumps and bumps. In my mind I hope for *moderate* but I always end up doing *active* or *challenging*! I guess I have my friends to thank for that!

Those last pushes on challenging days often make the most memorable moments. You don't necessarily want to push yourself too far... I heard of a man who cycled the Coast to Coast (140 miles) in a day then knocked himself out by falling over in the shower!

Nutrition

Nutrition and hydration are important. It would be unwise to think that you can cycle long distances without eating or drinking and it has been known for novice tourers to have Joan Collins moments - as in "You're not yourself when you're hungry!"

Get to know your body and energy needs. Through research or trial and error, you'll eventually discover what works best for you.

As a rough guide:

1. **Drink more water.** It's very easy to confuse dehydration with hunger so if you're hungry between meals try sipping water to fill the gap. You can add juice to your drink if you're going all day or it's hot but generally speaking, water will do. Replenish your bottles at every opportunity.

2. **Eat regularly.** Stick to a daily routine of three healthy meals - no junk, no meal replacements, no fads. Not eating properly won't help you lose weight any quicker (and it might make you fall off the bike). Some cyclists like to eat a

carb-heavy breakfast but make sure you leave enough time to digest your food before starting your ride.

3. **Carry emergency snacks.** Stock up on bananas and make your own trail mix/flapjack. Keep these in your jersey pockets so you won't need to stop to snack. It might be worth carrying an emergency energy gel in case you get lost or can't find the cafe for lunch. There's nothing worse than "bonking" and having no food on you.

As with any set of basic rules, disregard the ones that don't work for you!

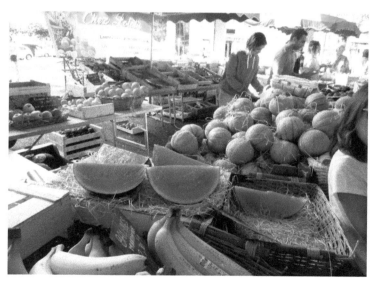

Fresh fruit from an outdoor farmers' market

Useful websites

Breeze - letsride.co.uk/breeze

Budget Cycling - budgetcycling.uk

Cycling UK - cyclinguk.org

Ruth McIntosh's blog on slow cycling - slow-cycle.com

Susan Doram's blog on her world tour - pfaffingandcycling.wordpress.com

Snjezana's business in Croatia - pintarska.com

Women's touring group, managed by Susan Doram and Joanne Westwood - facebook.com/groups/TotalWomenAwesomeTours

Acknowledgements

A special thanks to those who have held my hand, virtually speaking, during the process of writing: Susan Doram, Nicky Woods, Joanne Westwood, Lou Burkett, Alex Deck, Bev Kenyon, Chris Sissons, Glenda Strong, Douglas and Isobel McIntosh, Ellen McIntosh and Lisa Toffoletti.

Additional thanks to everyone who has supported me on Facebook.

About the Editor

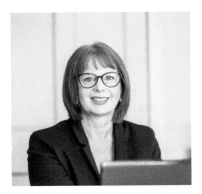

Ruth McIntosh: Editor, dreamer and slow-cyclist!

I started my blog www.slow-cycle.com after working as an English teacher for twenty years. I needed an escape... so writing about my love of cycle touring was an obvious choice!

After blogging alone in obscurity for a couple of years, I started to invite others to work with me on "Guest blogs." This helped me to discover that collaborative writing is great fun and the way forward! Now I use the writing methods that I have developed to offer Brand Storytelling for small businesses and not-for-profit organisations. Find out more and get in touch with me through my website: www.goodapplecopy.com.